YOUR KNOWLEDGE HAS VALUE

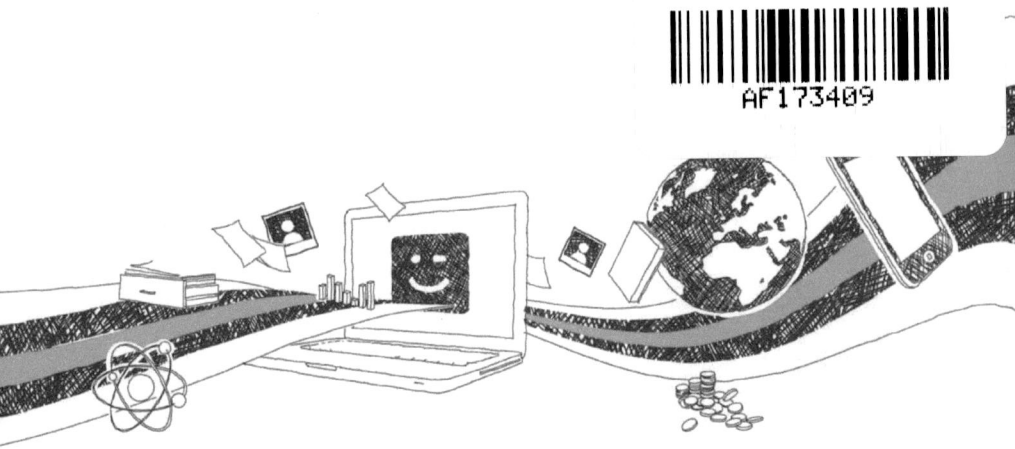
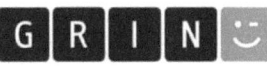

Bibliographic information published by the German National Library:

The German National Library lists this publication in the National Bibliography; detailed bibliographic data are available on the Internet at http://dnb.dnb.de .

Imprint:

Copyright © 2009 GRIN Verlag, Open Publishing GmbH
Print and binding: Books on Demand GmbH, Norderstedt Germany
ISBN: 9783640606849

This book at GRIN:

http://www.grin.com/en/e-book/149799/japan-health-elderly-and-child-care-in-comparison-to-the-german

Anja Hellmann

Japan: Health-, Elderly- and Child- Care in comparison to the German system: based on a case study

GRIN Publishing

GRIN - Your knowledge has value

Since its foundation in 1998, GRIN has specialized in publishing academic texts by students, college teachers and other academics as e-book and printed book. The website www.grin.com is an ideal platform for presenting term papers, final papers, scientific essays, dissertations and specialist books.

Visit us on the internet:

http://www.grin.com/

http://www.facebook.com/grincom

http://www.twitter.com/grin_com

Hochschule Bremen

Fakultät 3

Internationaler Studiengang für Pflege- und Gesundheitsmanagement (ISPG)

Japan:

Health-, Elderly- and Child- Care in comparison to the

German system: based on a case study

Studienarbeit

Semester*:*   *Sommersemester 2009*

Eingereicht von: *Anja Hellmann*

Contents

1 Introduction

The development of the Japanese society is characterized by a lot of similarities to Germany. This is why I have chosen the country to compare especially the Health Care System with the German one. Not only the economic achievements are comparable, but first of all the Demographic Change. In 2020 in Japan there will be 28% of the population over 65 years old. In Germany it is prognosticated to be around 21% (Tab.1). Moreover the Japanese Health Care System is known as own of the cheapest of the industrial countries. This leads to the question of adoption of some parts or ideas from the Japanese system to the German one. In my elaboration I want to describe a case of a family in Japan regarding the family and work situation, the Health Care System in general and additionally the system of taking care of the elderly and the children. My example family has got following parts: The mother is 42 years old, she works as a nurse in an outpatient department of a local government. In addition she has to take care of her parents almost every day. The father is 45 years old, works as an engineer and likes his hobby, which is driving motorbikes. The daughter of them is 7 and their son is 13, both go to school. The grandmother has got dementia, she is 76 years old and lives together with her husband, who is 76 and has got diabetes. They live in the neighborhood of their children and grandchildren.

Case 1: Values, Culture, roles of the family members.

Case 2: Health Care System of Japan in comparison to the German one. What happens after a traffic accident of the father?

Case 3: Elderly and Child Care in general and in the case of the accident and depression of the mother in the family.

2 Case 1

2.1 Home facilities/ Area where the family is living

In Japan the greater part of the population lives in the city (66%). A great part of the country is landscape, where it is not possible to occupy a house because it is really mountainous. This consequences the high density of population (340/km²) in comparison to Germany (236/km²).

One can imagine that this leads to the fact that a lot of people live in houses which are small and close to each other. Furthermore a lot of companies have their own houses for their workers (S.-C. Kim, 2005). Additionally there is great diversity between the social ranks. It is similar to the German situation. Because rich people get more and more money, whereas the middle class gets contemporary few money and is going to be minimized. The poverty of Japan is over the OECD average. Many people and first of all many children are poor and dependant on the welfare system. Nevertheless a lot of people in Japan are satisfied although belonging to a lower rank (S. Aßmann, 2004). The example family could belong to a middle rank. The father is a fully qualified and not an unlearned worker. And additional the mother works, what is nowadays more and more normal in Japan, but is not usual for a woman who has to take care of children and grandparents.

In the last decades there has been a great change in the lifestyle of the Japanese people. Consumption has become an important part of the society. This is caused by a long period of time where Japan was marked-out of the western world. The fact that people weren´t allowed to use all the achievements of the industrial nations and had a strict government leads to the extremity of usage of technical offers. It is used to show to which generation or group of thinking one belongs to. The isolation of oneself from the traditional way of thinking is very important for a lot of young people. (S. Aßmann, 2004). In the example family we would find traditional things, like Buddha, icons and pictures of their emperor next to the flat- screen, notebook and cell-phones.

2.2 Cultural values/ Religion

Many people have got a special picture of Japan in their head, which consists of: well- organized groups, Japanese copying other nations, too hard work, play little, travel around the world (J. Hendry, 2003). These are not false, but need to be defined. I want to give a short view of the culture of Japan which developed over a long time and with much influence: The culture of Japan is influenced by Russia, China and Europe. Most of the time there was a sys-

4

tem with social stratification and a strict regime. A major influence is given by the Chinese system and hereby first of all the Confucianism (J. Hendry, 2003).

At the beginning of the nineteenth century Japan was without influence of other nations or missioners. The nation developed extremely fast to a country with major power in the world. The economy grew and new technologies were find out by Japanese, whereas the self-consciousness grew (J. Hendry, 2003). Although there has been a change from a traditional to a more or less modern country the Japanese life is still influenced by rites and traditions. A main part of society is etiquette and the right behavior in all situations. Additionally religion plays a big role in the life of most of the people (J. Hendry, 2003). In year 2000 Shinto (108 million followers) and Buddhism (95.4 million followers) were the main religions as it was many hundred years ago. The whole population of Japan is only 127 million- what leads to the fact, that many people belong to more than only one religion. The example family would belong to both religions, too. They use the Shinto for their daily life. They pray to one of many gods for good grades, luck and visit their shrines. The Buddhism is used only for big happenings. Like the marriage of their children in some years or a funeral. Other minor religions are the Taoism, Confucianism and Christianity (J. Hendry, 2003).

2.3 Relationships/ Roles in the family

The system of family in Japan has been strengthened through the whole history. In cause of the extreme religions, like Confucianism, the roles in families have been the same for centuries. Just since the World War 2 the system changed slowly. Women became more rights and roles needed to be defined again. The Japanese call their family the "Ie", what means "house" or "family". This means not just the relatives, but all persons who have a great influence in life of one person. Even the dead and the unborn are included in this system and the Japanese think of them when they talk about the "Ie". A long time it was even written in the legal system, that people in one "Ie" were responsible for each other and had to take care of each other. (J. Hendry, 2003). This differs from our understanding to call only our direct relatives as our family.

2.3.1 Domestic situation

In the past it was also obligation to live in a house with all generations under one roof. So that the whole "Ie" was together. In the 80´s it was still typical to live with three generations in one house. Today the rate of people who live like this decreases as it does in other countries.

5

Many people live nowadays in a single-household or with a partner and children. The grandparents often live nearby, whereas the relatives still care for each other more than in other nations. The mother of our family has got responsibilities which are quite usual for Japanese circumstances. But even in Japan the number of people taking care of the elderly decreases (J. Hendry, 2003).

2.3.2 Male-Female Relations

Since 1946 the autonomy of the male is not guaranteed by law anymore. This means that women should have the same rights like the men. In reality a lot of things have already been changed, like the permission to work or the right of choice. But the roles still differ from each other. The men are often still the head of the family and earn the money. The Women are responsible for the budget, the children and elderly. Additionally many women have to work in a part- time job, because of the ailing economy and following decreasing salaries (50% of the married women work). In most parts of the society it is an ideal to have equal rights and for Japan it is even harder to reach this aim because of the traditions with their enormous influence (F. Coulmas, 2003).

2.3.3 Values of the family

The most important value for many Japanese is it to take care of their family in every situation, as it was mentioned before. Usually education of the children is another main part. All children enter school at the age of 6 officially, but a lot of them can read and write before. It is possible to give a child to the pre- school at the age of one and many people use this offer. At school children learn loyalty, there is a strict hierarchy between pupil and teacher and school endures mostly all-day and even on Saturdays. In 2002 there has been a reform , which indicates "to make education less regimented and more nurturing of children´s ability and willingness to solve problems by themselves" (J. Hendry, 2003, P.98). The third value is the company. To work for a company means to be deeply connected with it. For many people even company and their leaders are part of their family. Many work all their live in one and the same, they get the house from it, often the kindergartens and schools belong to it as well. Many firms have got an oath, a slogan and all have to wear the same cloth (F. Coulmas, 2003). Consumption is another value for many people. You need to have technical achievements and knowing about actual music, films etc. As I mentioned before the long period of time where Japan was isolated from the western world lead to a eagerness of new techniques and a feeling to be known as an industrial modern country as well (F. Coulmas, 2003). Other important values are the etiquette and the religion, which I have both described before.

3 Case 2

3.1 Health Care System of Japan

3.1.1 History

The Japanese government began in 1927 to provide a health insurance. This was focused on employees and not for elderly or people who were self-employed. In 1947 Japan was described as a welfare state by law. In the constitution a lower limit of healthy and cultured life was guaranteed. This also means that there were insurances against unemployment, for welfare, pension and of cause health care. In the case of the family mentioned at the beginning, one can say that after an accident of the father the family will get support by the welfare system comparable to Germany. Whereby the value of support won´t be that high as it is here in Germany, but basic support is guaranteed. In 1961 the health insurance for everyone was implemented. Nowadays the insurance is obligatory. When Japan implemented the first insurance, they orientated it quite close by the German Bismarck- model. In the following years the system worked well, but the rate of people over 65 grew and following in 1983 every insured had to pay a higher premium to ensure the supply of the elderly. Additionally since then people had to pay a part of the medical service privately.

In 1994 a reform implemented some new things in the system: more nurses in each hospital, higher additional payment by private, more ambulant services, private payment for the catering in the hospital (M. Schneider et al., 1994). In Germany we don´t have a fund for the elderly in the health care insurance like it is in Japan and we don´t have so many and high additional amounts. Another big difference in the system are the private insurances. The Japanese don´t have it because they want the system to be as equal as possible.

3.1.2 Insurances

In total there are more than 5000 independent insurance plans in Japan, which can be divided in three parts: The first plan is an insurance for large- firm employees and their dependants, which is called the "Society – Managed Health Insurance". For the public- sector employees it is called "Mutual Aid Associations". They have to pay 6%- 9.5% of monthly wages. Employer and employee pay each the half of it. The second plan is the insurance for small- firm employees (Government- Managed Health Insurance), which is operated by the Ministry of Health and Welfare. Here the premium is about 8.6 % and the employee pays the half of it.

Dependants are family- insured in the first and second plan, even if there is only a cohabitation. The third plan is for self- employed and pensioners (Citizens´ Health Insurance), which is operated by all the 3000 cities, towns and villages in Japan. The premium is based on the income, number of people living in household and assets (N. Ikegami, J. C. Campbell, 1999).

3.1.3 Financing System

The system is financed by the premiums, subsidies of the government and additional private payment by the insured, which differ from 10-30% depending on age and revenue. In 1998 the premiums made 52.9%, the additional payment 14.9% and the government paid with taxes 32.2%. Although the system is subsidized by the government, 70% of the insurances made a deficit in 1999, whereas most of them are insurances for people with a low income (H. Jeong, 2001). The main difference to Germany is the high rate of subsidies. If these were not, the Health Care System of Japan wouldn´t seem to be so cheap. Moreover the system differs at the rate of private payment. In Germany we have to pay for service mainly 10€ every three months and of course for special services (IGE- Leistungen). In Japan you have to pay for every service and additionally the whole catering in hospital. In general you can say the services for which the insurance pays are quite similar to the German system, including Rehabilitation and sick- payment. But in all cases, even in the case of emergency you have to pay from private up to a special rate each month (around 400 €). Mainly in the psychotherapeutically sector many long- term- therapies are not included in the insurance, what goes together with the fact that psychological illnesses are still a taboo in Japanese society and these illnesses are expensive and hard to bear for those people (Sonnenmoser, M., 2008).

3.1.4 Hospitals and doctors

In Japan one can choose to go to a physician´s office or to the hospital directly. All of the doctors are in solo-practices and they often (1/3 of them) have some beds and are called clinics. If someone has got more than 20 beds these are hospitals. All of the clinics and hospitals have got many beds for the ambulant patients. Nowadays many hospitals still have long- term patient beds next to the beds for acute patients. But more and more homes for the elderly are built and so this seems to change. This system differs a lot to the German one. Here it is not possible to go to hospital without an assignment and long- term and acute beds are separated strictly. Similar to Germany is, that the private hospitals are smaller than the public- sector hospitals (N. Ikegami, 1999). In Japan all clinics and hospitals were paid identically a long time. After the reform in 2000 the system turned away from the fee- for- service payment. They thought about the DRG system as it works in many other countries in the world. But they decided to implement the Diagnosis and Procedure Combination (DPC), which pays the hospital for each day plus fee- for-service if the patient stays longer than he should. The DRG system in Germany pays only for each day in a special period of time for each illness. In Japan it is a problem that only 10% of all hospitals are coding with ICD, which is the requirement for the DPC (N. Ikegami, 2002).

3.1.5 Costs for services

In Japan the costs are lower because of many facts, which are cause by the culture and behavior of the people. The rates of crime, divorce, teenage births, drug use, accidents and the incidence of HIV are lower than in comparable countries. Furthermore the living habits and nutrition are much better, what may contribute to better health. Heart- diseases are much more rarely than in Germany. Another point is that Japanese have a cultural antipathy for invasive procedures and like to use the conservative way of treatment. And in addition the fees for surgery are really low and here the costs normally would be really high. In general the government controls all the costs in the Health Care System. The fees for high-tech treatments are low and the one for ordinary consultations, laboratory test, diagnostics and medicine are higher (N. Ikegami, 1999). In 2002 the prices of medical services and for drugs were cut by an average of 2.7% (N. Ikegami, 2002). In Germany the structure is conversely. High- technology and surgery cost a lot and the fees are higher therefore as for ordinary services. As I already explained the system in Japan is weighted on outpatient care, so that Japan "has the highest rate of physician visits and the lowest rate of hospital admissions among advanced industrial nations" (N. Ikegami, 1999, S. 60). Additionally the practicing doctors in 1999 had a rate of 1.9 doctor per 1000 of population. In Germany there are 3.4 doctors per 1000. Japan lays under the OECD average of 2.9 doctors per 1000 of population in 1999 (Tab 2). On the other hand Japan has got more beds in hospitals and clinics than the OECD average- what can be explained by a lot of beds which are used for long- term- patients and from 1990 on the number of beds decreases in Japan, too.

One fact is quite remarkable: The length of stay in hospital is the highest of all OECD countries. In 1999 in Japan the average was about 30.8 days. The average of all OECD countries is about 7-8%. The long-term patient beds are one reason for this. Another is for example too many beds built in the 80´s and the hospitals wanted to fill them. The third reason is "social hospitalization". People used the hospitals to have someone who cared for the relatives for some weeks- whereas homes for the elderly for long or short time weren´t built in such a high number (H. Jeong, 2002).

3.1.6 Problems and aims

Like many other countries Japans Health Care System suffers in cause of the Demographic Change. Five major problems become more and more apparent: growing consumer consciousness, a rapidly aging population, rising costs, inequality of burden and quality of care:First, people are more conscious and want to have detailed information by the physicians. Ethical questions become more important and the relationship between patient and provider needs to be changed, otherwise the confidence will decrease.

Secondly the aging population costs a lot, because they need more medical supply and care institutions. And simultaneously less children are born, who would once be able to pay for the system. In April 2000 the government implemented the long- term care insurance program, which is orientated on the German system.

The third and most serious problem are the costs, which rise through the Demographic Change, but also because the downturn of the economy. People don´t earn so much money and therefore premiums become lower. Additionally people pay less taxes , which are an important part of the financing system. At least in 2002 prices for medical services and drugs were reduced again by the government by an average of 2.7 %. Moreover they wanted to change the payment system into DPC (Diagnosis and Procedure Combinations), but only 10% of hospitals are able to implement, because 90% don´t even code with ICD- system. Moreover there are too many beds in hospitals and people stay too long at hospital (Tab 3).

Another point is the difference in the financial health of insurers. Some of them won´t be able to exist a long time anymore, because of the differences of insured people. They think about risk adjustment regarding age, sex and illnesses as it is just done in Germany. Finally the quality of care is a big problem. There is no external evaluation of hospitals or other services. Professional protocols are not usual and many buildings are run- down , rooms are crowded and there is a deficit of support staff . A solution could be to change the payment system, implement accreditation, quality management, the differentiation between long- term care and acute beds and create a competition. These are the big problems of the health care System in Japan and many a quite similar to German problems, whereas Germany has already done a lot more to solve these problems, especially regarding the evaluation, competition and quality management (N. Ikegami, 1999).

4 Case 3

4.1 Elderly Care

4.1.1 Demographic Change

Comparable to almost every other industrialized country, Japan´s Demographic Change affects the Health Care System a lot. In 2005 20% of the population of Japan are over the age of 65. In 2020 they are going to represent 28% of the population. In Germany the rate rises from 18% (2005) to 21% (2020) (Tab 1). Moreover the birth rate of Japan is declining more than in most of the other industrial nations (Botschaft von Japan). As a conclusion the number of population shrinks and the population becomes older on average. In addition the life expectancy in Japan is one of the highest in the world (S.- C. Kim, 2005).

4.1.2 The "Gold plans"

The importance of the Demographic Change was realized and discussed first in the 80´s. In 1989 the so called "Gold plan" was set in. It included a ten year strategy to Promote Health Care and Welfare for the elderly. Welfare offices were built and social workers started their work in collaboration with volunteers to understand the situation of the elderly and show how to change the situation of taking care of them. Day service centers, nursing homes for elderly and group homes for elderly with dementia were built. In 1994 the "New Gold plan" was established. It included a higher number of helpers for the homes for elderly and the capacities of short- stay facilities was improved. Additionally the at- home service with doctors and nurses was enlarged. Until this point of time an organized system for elderly care was appointed, but it didn´t reach the majority of people seeking for help. And people who needed a long- term care were not provided. In 2000 the "Gold plan 21" got started. This included an insurance system for long- term care. It was leaned on the German system of insurance. The "Gold plan 21" contains long- term care services, measures for senile people, measures to revitalize the elderly and a support system in communities (Web Japan, Fact Sheet, http://web-japan.org/factsheet/pdf/41Welfare.pdf).

4.1.3 The long- term care insurance system

The long- term care insurance is similar to the German one, but some differences are noticeable. The premium in Germany is fixed and paid by every person who pays for the health care insurance, in Japan the local communities define how much to pay and only people over the age of 40 have to pay. Additionally in Japan there are five levels for the need of care and people get more money than in Germany (Tab 4), but hey only get non- cash benefits, like professional care. Moreover people who need help have to pay about 10% from private assets and only people over the age of 65 get help whereas in Germany everyone gets help who is rated in one of the three levels of need (S. Shimada, 2006). Moreover in Japan Care-Manager are involved in the system of the insurance. They are the connecting part between the elderly, their families and the insurances on the other side. Every person gets an individual plan of care, which is elaborated by the Care- Manager. In Germany the family decides more less alone what services they occupy (S. Shimada, 2006).

The financing of the long- term care system is taken by the national government (25%), the local government (about 12.5%), the insurance premiums (50%) and by private (10%) (Web Japan, Fact Sheet, http://web-japan.org/factsheet/pdf/41Welfare.pdf).

Nowadays the government tries to focus on home care services instead of long- term services as it is in Germany, too, because costs are far smaller. And another comparable point is the importance of prevention to minimize costs in future.

The family, mentioned at the beginning of my work, has got the opportunity to use an home-care service to take care of the grandmother with dementia and to ensure the supply of the grandfather with diabetes. On the other hand they could choose an short- time care or day-service centers. In every case the grandparents need to be raged in a level of need of care and then they will get a Care- Manager who will provide them with professional advice.

4.2 Child Care

Contemporary to the implementation of the health care insurance in 1947, the Child Welfare Law became legally valid. It involved the opening of child guidance centers in Japan with specially educated child welfare workers. They advise the parents, when they need it and they are authorized to organize a foster family for children. Additionally the local welfare offices and health centers employ volunteers and social workers, who support children, pregnant women and mothers who need assistance. There are some facilities for the child care, like homes for infants, day nurseries, support centers for households with children and hospital homes for children with disabilities. In 1995 the "Angel Plan" was implemented this was an 10- year agenda for the expansion of the capacity of all institutions for children with the aim of increasing the birth rate by making it possible for women to work and have children. In 1999 the "New Angel plan" involved again more various types of care facilities and 2003 the prevention got more important to bring up healthy children. In general one can say, that all these implementations helped many mothers to work and have a family, but at the end the birth rate still decreases and this couldn´t be stopped through all innovations in the system of child care (Web Japan, Fact Sheet). In the case of our family, the children could be looked after by one of the various types of day care or by a foster family if it is necessary. On the other hand children are often all day at school and need help only in the evening and during the night.

5 Conclusion

In general one can say, that Japan is a welfare state, where all the insurances are implemented as they are in Germany. But after a deeper look it is obvious that people of the middle class are not able to pay all the private additional amounts, which would be necessary in the case of the family, mentioned in the introduction, after the father had an accident and the mother a depression. For every service of medical care an additional amount would be relevant (30%) up to a special number every month, the service for the grandparents is taken with 10% by private and the children care needed to be paid, too. With the look at this example it gets obvious, that the care for all of the family- members is not able to be financed. The "Ie", which is the whole family and close friends still plays a big role in the Japanese society. It is needed for the supply for all family members, which is not taken by the community as much as it is in Germany. A lot of people in Japan can´t pay their bills for medical service anymore nowadays. In this special case of the family it could be really difficult for them, too, depending on their assets and their family system, which could be a great support.

The system in Japan is much cheaper than the German one, but on the other hand the supply is not as comprehensive as it is in Germany and many people cannot afford a great part of the service in Japan. And in every case it is harder for the Japanese to get social benefit than it is in Germany.

6 List of literature

Anonym (2005) *Große Besorgnis über sinkende Geburtenrate in Japan; kein Ende des Trends in Sicht.* [online]. Berlin, Foreign press Center Japan. Einsehbar unter: http://www.de.emb-japan.go.jp/presse/nochnicht/jb_050610.htm [Stand 05. Mai.2009].

Aßmann, S. (2004) *Wertewandel und soziale Schichtung in Japan: Differenzierungsprozesse im Konsumenten-verhalten japanischer Frauen.* Hamburg, Institut für Asienkunde.

Coulmas, F. (2003) *Die Kultur Japans: Tradition und Moderne.* München, Verlag C.H. Beck oHG

Hendry, J. (2003) *Understanding Japanese Society.* Third Edition. New York, Routledge/Curzon.

Ikegami, N. und Campbell, J.- C. (1999). Health Care Reform In Japan: The Virtues Of Muddling Through. *Health Affairs: The Policy Journal of the Health Sphere,* 18 (3), S. 56-75. Full- text [online]. Health Affairs [Stand 05.Mai 2009].

Ikegami, N. und Campbell, J.- C. (2004). Japan´s Health Care System: Containing Costs And Attempting Re-form. *Health Affairs: The Policy Journal of the Health Sphere,* 23 (3), S. 26- 36. Full- text [online]. Health Affairs [Stand 05.Mai 2009].

Japan Fact Sheet (undatiert) *Health Care: Aiming for high- quality and sustainable health and medical services.* [online]. Einsehbar unter: http://web-japan.org/factsheet/pdf/42Healthcare.pdf [Stand 05. Mai 2009].

Japan Fact Sheet (undatiert) *Welfare: Helping the elderly, the young, and the disabled.* [online]. Einsehbar unter: http://web-japan.org/factsheet/pdf/41Welfare.pdf [Stand 05. Mai 2009].

Kim, S.-C. (2005) *„Unternehmenszentrierte Gesellschaft" und Sozialstaat in Japan.* Frankfurt am Main, Euro-päischer Verlag der Wissenschaften.

Rebick, M. und Takenaka, A. (2006) *The Changing Japanese family.* New York, Routledge.

Schneider, M. und Biene- Dietrich, P. (1994) Japan. *In: Gesundheitssysteme im internetionalen Vergleich.* Augsburg, BASYS. S. 313- 331

Shimada, S. und Tagsold, C. (2006) *Alternde Gesellschaft im Vergleich: Solidarität und Pflege in Deutschland und Japan.* Bielefeld, transcript Verlag.

Sonnenmoser, M. (2008) Zwischen Tradition und westlichen Einflüssen. *Deutsches Ärzteblatt* [online], 2008 (6). Einsehbar unter: http://aerzteblatt.lnsdata.de/pdf/PP/7/6/s264.pdf

Stitzel, A., Buchner, F., Janig, H. (2008) *Pflegeversicherungen im Vergleich: Deutschland und Japan.* Wien, Hauptverband der österreichischen Sozialversicherungsträger.

List of tables

Tab 1:

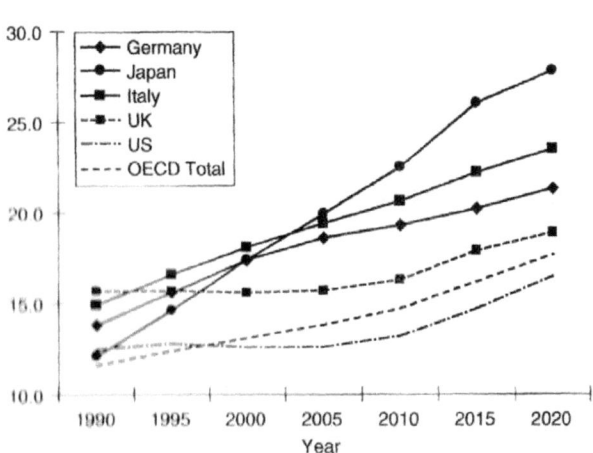

Figure 1.1 Percentage of population over age 65, selected OECD countries.
Source: United Nations, Population Database.

15

Tab 2:

Chart 9: Practising doctors* per 1000 population

(in 1999)

Turkey	1.2
Korea	1.3
Mexico	1.7
United Kingdom	1.8
Japan**	1.9
Canada	2.1
Poland	2.3
New Zealand	2.3
Ireland	2.3
Australia**	2.5
United States**	2.7
Norway	2.8
France**	3
Czech Republic	3
Austria	3
Sweden	3.1
Spain	3.1
Netherlands	3.1
Luxembourg	3.1
Finland	3.1
Portugal	3.2
Hungary	3.2
Iceland**	3.3
Switzerland	3.4
Germany**	3.4
Denmark	3.4
Belgium	3.8
Greece**	4.2
Italy	5.9

Doctors per 1000 population

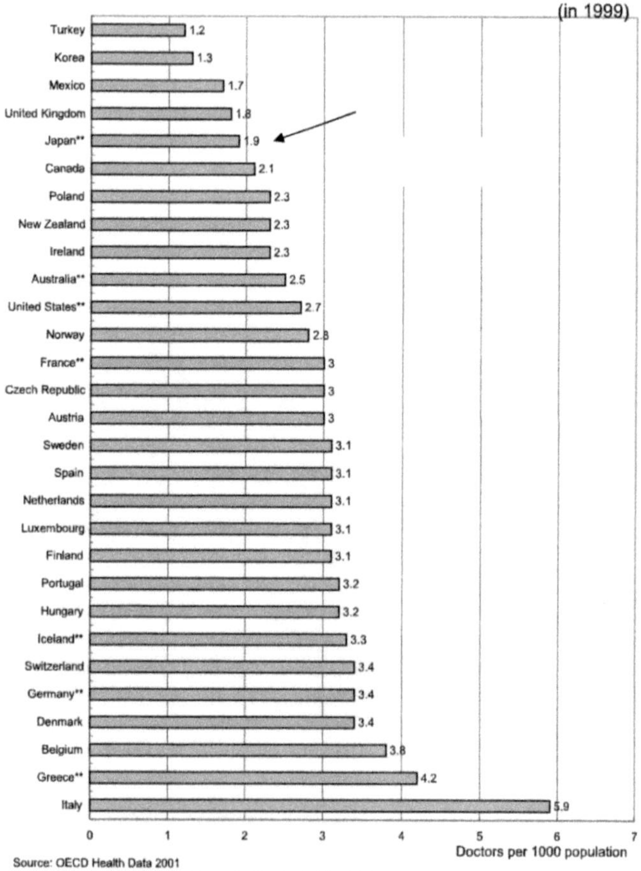

Source: OECD Health Data 2001
*Data for Finland Italy and Spain are physicians entitled to practice
** Data are for 1998

16

Tab 3:

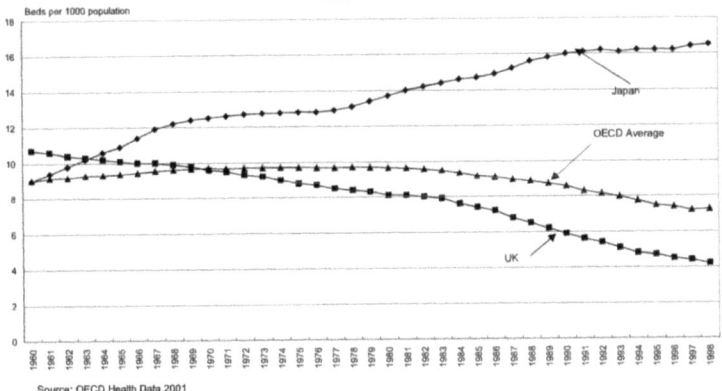

Chart 10: Trends in number of beds in inpatient care facilities per 1000 population,
1960-1998

Source: OECD Health Data 2001

Tab 4:

Monthly output per benefit recipient:

Monatliche Leistungsausgabe je Leistungsempfänger

	Japan * (EUR)	Deutschland ** (EUR)
ambulant	750	540
stationär	3.038	1.259 ***

* Im November 2002
** Durchschnittswert im Jahr 2000
*** Vollstationäre Pflege

Source/ Quelle: Ministerium für Arbeit, Gesundheit und Wohlfahrt
Bundesministerium für Gesundheit, Statistisches Taschenbuch
2001
Bundesministerium für Arbeit und Sozialordnung, Bundesarbeitsblatt
4/2001

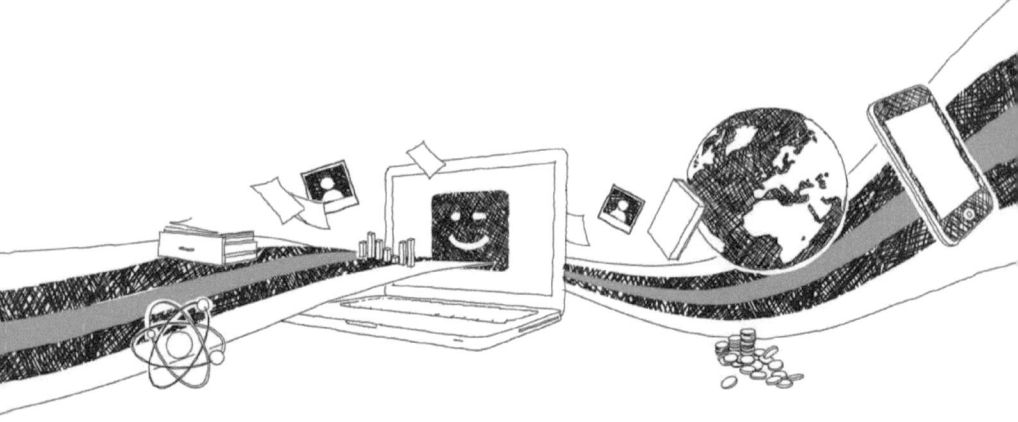
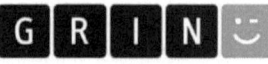